Body Reset Diet

Speed Up Your Metabolism, Burn Fat & Lose Weight Quickly!

Keith Alexander

Table of Contents

Legal Disclaimer

The information contained in this book is strictly for educational purpose only. The content of this book is the sole expression and opinion of its author and not necessarily that of the publisher. It is not intended to cure, treat, and diagnose any kind of disease or medical condition. It is sold with the understanding that the publisher is not rendering any type of medical, psychological, legal, or any other kind of professional advice. You should seek the services of a competent professional before applying concepts in this book. Neither the publisher nor the individual author(s) shall be liable for any physical, psychological, emotional, financial, or commercial damages, directly or indirectly by the use of this material, which is provided "as is", and without warranties. Therefore, if you wish to apply ideas contained in this book, you are taking full responsibility for your actions.

Introduction

You've probably tried a plethora of various diets and they just haven't worked. Or maybe they did, at first, but now you've reached a plateau and you just can't seem to get rid of those last five pounds. Maybe you've become a chronic dieter, managing to stick to a certain diet for just a couple of days and then falling off track only to start again a while later, but with no fruitful results.

You've been hitting the gym and keeping a close eye on that scale but somehow it just never seems to show you what you want to see. So if you're looking for a quick, effective, revolutionary way of losing weight, this book will show you how.

So stop feeling disappointed if your previous diets haven't worked for you. The body reset diet will change the way you look at weight loss!

For years, people have followed different diet loss fads that came and went, and none was considered quite a breakthrough when it came to weight loss. Most of them just consisted of difficult to follow, complicated diet plans that not only left a person feeling hungry and undernourished, but most people fell off the wagon soon enough.

Even worse, when you do finally manage to lose a few pounds, you gain it all back by going back to your old ways. We've all gone through at least one such experience. Whether it involves starving yourself or training hours at the gym, the end result is the same. So what exactly have we been doing wrong all this time and how exactly do we counter past failures and do it right this time around?

This is where the body reset diet comes in. We have trained our bodies, unfortunately, to be dependent on the fatty, unhealthy foods that are part of our everyday routine. So obviously, when we take that food away, all of a sudden our body is not used to it at all!

The body reset diet, however, is not just about cutting down on calories. It's about unlearning old dietary habits and training our bodies to learn new ones. We train our bodies to get used to a low-calorie, high energy diet that prompts our system to switch to fat-burning mode. The idea behind this diet is for people to stick to a diet that gives them fast results instead of leaving them feeling drained. People all over the world are testing out the body rest diet, with favorable results, so don't miss out this chance at a life-changing opportunity, and learn how to reset your body now!

1: What Is Body Reset Diet?

The main focus of this diet is to basically boost your metabolism and reset your system in a way that you reboot your entire body to set yourself on the trajectory to sustained weight loss and good health.

This diet consists of getting the bulk of your nutrients from smoothies, soups and minor snacks for the first five days, and then slowly easing your body back into eating solid food over the next period of days. It has an 'eat more, weigh less' theory to it. By increasing the meals, but making them low calorie and high in nutrition, you will manage to starve off hunger and also lose weight.

The duration of this metabolic reset depends on you alone. If you feel that it is benefiting and you want to keep losing those extra pounds, then you can continue it for however long you want, without any health risks involved.

Every other traditional diet out there helps you lose weight but only while you're on the diet. The minute you revert back to your usual eating style, you pack on all that weight all over again. In addition, the results are slow to achieve and possibly not what you expected. Body Reset Diet will help you kick your metabolism into high gear and restart it.

As we age, most of us experience much slower metabolism than before. They find themselves either gaining weight or struggling to lose weight, which is why usual diets don't work as effectively as the entire system has just slowed down.

However, when you boost your metabolism rate, this helps your body start burning those calories much faster and allows you to have higher energy levels than normal. By making changes to how often you eat and what you eat, you can make a huge difference. That's all that there is to it. The secret to weight loss as explained by this diet is simple, it's not just about what you eat, but it's also about your timing.

We've trained ourselves to keep producing constant amount of hormones that promote hunger and thus we keep craving food throughout the day. By doing this, we're caught in a "fat cycle", and by tuning into the needs of our body's natural routine, we can break out of this cycle and finally say goodbye to the extra pounds.

The success of this diet is the fact that it lays the foundation for a healthy lifestyle. People who follow a strict weight loss lifestyle are much more capable of not only reaching their goal weight but also maintaining their weight in the long run.

So what exactly is the Body Reset Diet? It is a fifteen day plan and it is separated into three phases. During the first phase you are supposed to only have smoothies as meals. In the second phase, you are supposed to drink two smoothies and replace one of the smoothies with food like a sandwich or stir fry.

In the last phase, you switch two smoothies and have full meals instead. Going to the gym isn't recommended on this diet either; all the diet suggests is that one must walk around ten thousand steps a day. You may also do some light resistance training about three times a week. This diet is guaranteed to help you lose weight fast, but how quickly will that happen depend on you alone.

While some may worry that there might be some associated health risks, this is not the case. However, it is advisable that before making any major changes in your diet, you should always consult with your doctor.

Unlike other diets, this diet does not promote starving yourself to lose weight. In fact, it adheres pretty well to the accepted dietary guidelines:

FAT - You should stay in the accepted recommendation of twenty to thirty-five percent of daily fat intake. In fact, a sample menu will generally be around twenty-three percent.

PROTEIN - The diet is also in the normal range of protein intake. The recommended value is ten to thirty-five percent and this diet provides you with twenty-two percent of protein.

CARBOHYDRATES - It is advised to get about forty-five to sixty five percent of your daily calories in the form of carbohydrates. The Body Reset Diet will maintain around sixty-two percent.

In addition, this diet is also very easy to follow. It emphasizes the need to be satisfied and feel full after every meal, which is why it is so successful. A wide variety of delicious smoothies also makes phase 1 easy and enjoyable. Thus, this diet helps boost your metabolism and kick start your path to weight loss in an easy, effective way.

2: The Benefits – Why Go For Body Reset?

The first few days of this diet consist of mainly smoothies and soups. That means that most of your nutrition is plant-based, and it is not only low in calories but also very high in energy.

However, in all honestly, the idea of giving up solid food sounds pretty intimidating. What exactly does this strategy have to offer when it comes to resetting your metabolism? Well, the first benefit of this diet is based not on what you're eating but what you AREN'T eating.

The wide variety of unhealthy, processed, high sugar and high fat food that we eliminate during the body rest allows our body to take a break from all the work involved in digesting these foods.

It is our dietary habits that make us feel lethargic and unhealthy. Instead, we replace these foods with high fiber and low-calorie smoothies that are rich in micronutrients. Ninety-five percent of the vitamins and enzymes that our body needs are found in the juice of raw vegetables and fruits.

One sixteen ounce of fresh juice gives us more nutrients than consuming large amounts of the same fruits and vegetables. Thus, these smoothies are more efficient and much faster in getting our share of the highly concentrated enzymes, vitamins, and minerals.

This change in diet from high sugar, high calorie, to low calorie, high in fiber foods not only help detoxify the body but it sets the body on the path to weight loss by burning fat, instead of continuously storing it inside of our bodies.

ENERGY

Resetting your body means switching to a high energy, healthy diet that initially involves just having smoothies. Extracted from fruits and vegetables, they are packed with antioxidants, minerals, and also vitamins. Smoothies are a concentrated form of all these amazing nutritional components. Once these natural sugars and micronutrients enter the bloodstream and the level of glucose rises, you can definitely feel the surge in energy from all the nutrients pumped into your body.

IMMUNITY

Research shows that people with well-balanced healthy dietary lifestyles are much less prone to disease and illness, especially given that you will be incorporating various smoothies into your diet. For example, vegetables like bok choy and broccoli contains specific compound that is greatly beneficial to the immune system. They provide another layer of protection against various cells in the human body against invasion. Thus, going on a metabolism reset diet positively affects other systems in the body too by up-regulating them to be stronger and more efficient.

NUTRITIONAL BENEFIT

Apart from the effect that the body reset has on your metabolism, the nutritional benefits it provides are endless. This diet will result in your food being an excellent source of anti-oxidants which are absolutely indispensable to the body. In the everyday metabolic functions of the body, natural process is always ongoing.

This is the production of 'free radicals' inside the body. This is a by-product of body metabolism and the production of energy. Even though this is a naturally occurring process, it is not without consequence. Free radicals are highly toxic to body tissues and are capable of causing wide-spread and extensive damage to body tissues. This is where anti-oxidants are important and play their role. These antioxidants remove free radicals from the body system, aiding in the process of detoxification.

Science now proves that a high anti-oxidant intake is useful in preventing a number of life threatening, and possibly terminal diseases. These included various cancers and even Alzheimer's. Furthermore, the physical manifestations are clearly written on your skin.

The skin becomes rejuvenated and more vibrant, and antioxidants also prevent further wrinkles and skin damage in the future. Some very commonly known anti-oxidant include Vitamin A, C, and E. The body reset diet will help incorporate these same vitamins and anti-oxidants into your own diet.

Vitamin C is invaluable in skin and gum health, whereas vitamin A is also vital for the eyes and skin. Apart from the abundance of antioxidants that you will receive as part of the body reset diet, there a number of other essential nutrients that are packed in the healthy foods you will be incorporating. Some examples include:

FOLIC ACID

Folic acid is absolutely vital for the human body. Green smoothies and leafy green vegetables are one of the best known sources. A deficiency of folic acid can lead to severe anemia. In pregnancy, folic acid deficiency in the mother can be absolutely devastating to the developing baby in the first trimester of pregnancy, resulting in severe defects in the development of the neural tube. Thus, pregnant women are specifically advised to increase their intake of folic acid.

POTASSIUM

Potassium is important for electrolyte regulation inside the human body. An adequate intake of potassium helps the heart and kidney to function properly and make them healthy and efficient. In addition, potassium helps the muscles maintain their strength and also aids the nervous system to work properly. When potassium intake is low, you may feel exhausted, dizzy, muscle aches and pains, along with chronic headaches. A more serious deficiency can also lead to palpitations.

VITAMIN A

Apart from the benefits of vitamin A as an effective antioxidant, it is especially important to be able to see at night. Lack of vitamin A can result in night blindness. Furthermore, it also prevents macular degeneration in the elderly.

VITAMIN C

Vitamin C is indispensable for the proper tissue development and functioning of the skin and the gums. A deficiency of vitamin C can eventually lead to scurvy, a disease which results in bleeding of gums.

FIBER

One of the most important reasons why the body reset diet is so effective is because of the high fiber intake associated with this diet. Since fiber is insoluble and can remains undigested through the intestines and the digestive system, it helps to regulate bowel functioning.

Furthermore, it also aids in the softening of stool that eases the intestine's work and making digestion easier. The fiber that remains undigested lowers cholesterol levels by trapping all the fat and cholesterol in the diet, which in turn prevents cholesterol absorption and leads to a healthy heart. Increased fiber intake also makes you feel full, which helps ward off hunger and cravings for unhealthy food. This in turn will help you lose weight.

Resetting your metabolism also involves low cholesterol intake. The body reset diet can help drastically bring down unhealthy cholesterol. High levels of bad cholesterol in the body cause deposition of this same cholesterol in the arteries and vessels. As time passes, this deposition causes narrowing of the vessels eventually causing a complete occlusion. This could eventually result in an embolism, heart attack or even stroke by cutting off circulation to the brain.

Another benefit body reset diet is the increased levels of hydration in the body. It is imperative to have as much water as possible, even up to three liters a day. Dehydration is a common cause of fatigue, decreased cognitive functioning, and headaches. You start this diet by consuming only smoothies and liquids. Solid foods are not allowed during consumption of smoothies, soups, and water throughout the day as the body needs to remains well hydrated. Good hydration leads to glowing, younger looking skin as it flushes out toxins from the system making the cells healthier.

The healthy diet plan that the body reset diet recommends is also rich in *Phytonutrients* that are found in natural foods like vegetables. These phytonutrients are very useful to the body. It can prevent cancers in the colon, pancreas, breast and urinary bladder. The body reset diet also helps keep diabetes in check. The low sugar content efficiently keeps sugar and insulin levels in check. This helps the pancreatic functioning in the long run and prevents the development of diseases that may result secondary to diabetes.

BENEFITS OF ALKALINITY

Most of our food intake leaves our bodies acidic. Animal-based foods and processed foods all contribute to this. This is why body reset is so beneficial to our body. It promotes alkalinity that helps make us feel content and more energetic whereas an acidic body makes us feel more depressed and tired. Filling your body with vibrant, fresh foods will help you keep the body alkaline and make you feel more balanced and flexible. In case you have too much alkaline in your diet, our dietary constituents always help balance it out.

3: Detoxification during the Body Reset

Most people get nervous when they hear the term detoxification, even though there is no reason to. When undertaking the body reset diet, you are adopting a new food pattern that will pave the way for a healthy lifestyle. This is why this diet is so effective. It offers an amalgamation of all the benefits of a healthy diet in addition to weight loss. It's not just about keeping your weight in check by metabolism reset, but this reset cleanses your body to make you feel healthy and energetic.

When done correctly, body reset and detoxification are just different words to describe a healthy, nutritious diet that is rich in natural, raw, unprocessed whole foods. When you remove the artificial flavors and chemicals from your daily dietary intake, this helps re-set your body and make your body healthier. By getting rid of the all the negative influences on your diet, you can extract the benefits of healthy foods that will help you lose weight fast.

How exactly does a body reset stimulate your body to detoxify itself? The principle of this diet is to kick start your system by just having all natural smoothies for the first five to ten days. These smoothies, consisting of different enzymes and made of raw food help the body to get into action.

This helps convert the body into a cleaning house of sorts. It starts by getting rid of old body cells, removing debris from the organs and tissues, and transitioning into creating new, healthy cells, and thus a much healthier body.

It is due to this reason that some people prefer not to switch too abruptly from their normal diet to a body reset diet plan. By switching too early, it can cause an array of uncomfortable symptoms as a result of the detoxification.

During the detoxification process the different cells of the body purge themselves of metabolic waste alongside different environmental toxins. It end up releasing them into the bloodstream so that they may be transported to the liver and kidneys; finally being removed from the body.

Once all the toxic and waste material are exposed to these organs, the organs start excreting as much of this same material out of the body so the bowels, lungs, kidneys, liver and even the skin start to get rid of their waste through stool, urine, sweat and even through menstruation in females. A lot of these toxins are also excreted through the mucous in the throat and sinuses.

Even in normal everyday routine, the body is constantly trying to eliminate toxins and waste products in the body. However, our dietary habits have become so unnatural that we put our body through a constant attack by overeating, stress, and chemicals.

For this reason, the body cannot function as efficiently in its effort to get rid of all the waste. Its capacity to function at its best is greatly diminished. Over time, there is a gradual increase in toxins in the tissues and in the bowels. This causes a much quicker process of aging, illness, and fatigue. In some cases, this might also be the reason for obesity and inability to lose weight.

Thankfully, the body is quite equipped to heal itself, and it is a methodical machine persistently trying to maintain a perfect balance in the body and promoting wellness. A constant system of removal of toxins and waste is always ongoing, and it is believed that during this process of elimination the body tends to undergo some 'symptoms' of detoxification.

Detoxification is a process of self-purification that is ongoing at all times, but it is most effective in the morning. Thus, it is beneficial to start the day right with a healthy breakfast smoothie early in the morning. If you kick start your morning with heavy food, it will prolong this same process, and in some cases, causes a person to stay obese and overweight.

This phase of detoxification is also known as a 'catabolic phase' as the body is destroying unhealthy cells only to replace them later with healthier ones. By repairing the damage caused by our habits, it is now ready to progress to the 'anabolic' phase of rebuilding.

The body is provided with all that is needed to keep functioning in a healthy and pure manner on the inside, but our dietary choices can greatly speed up this process. This is the role that the body reset plays to help you lose weight. There is no need to spend your time and money on different products that claim to aid weight loss, like saunas or devices because they play no role in regulating the internal body functions and are thus are useless.

In addition to detoxification, the body also works on repairing the damage and ensuring that new cells are developed. During this process, the body requires more rest than usual as this repair usually occurs while we sleep.

When this phase begins, it is expected that one needs more rest for the healing process to take place. It is best that we appreciate this process of healing and do everything possible to aid it. During the first few day of your body reset diet, it is advisable that you take a break from all energy-consuming activities as this will retract the main goal of your body reset.

The more you rest and relax, the more your body will focus on detoxifying itself. The best gift we can give to ourselves is allowing the body to reboot itself so it can work more efficiently.

4: Starting the Body Reset

There are three main phases to the body reset diet, with each one lasting about five days each. Ideally, you have to start losing weight the day you begin this diet.

In all three stages of this diet, you must eat five times a day, no more, no less. You need to train your body to get used to set timings. In the first phase, you will only have smoothies three times a day and two snacks in a day. In the second phase, one smoothie is replaced by a low-calorie meal and then in the third phase two of these smoothies are replaced by a low-calorie meal. Then you can gradually ease yourself back into your normal eating routine.

The first phase, which involves an all-liquid diet, is the part that most people struggle with, due to food cravings plus withdrawal systems and symptoms of detoxification of the body.

However, this is the part that boosts your metabolism. It is very important you stick through this part of the diet without faltering. Once you make it through the first couple of days, you will feel your energy skyrocket. While you are on this diet, the goal is to leave you feeling content so you won't be tempted towards unhealthy snacking.

If you have any health concerns before starting the body reset diet, then do consult your doctor. If you're on any medication, remember to consult with your doctor to see whether you should keep taking it. First and foremost, before undergoing any dietary changes, it is always best to consult with your medical practitioner.

The first couple of days of reset are the hardest for most people. This is when the body is undergoing withdrawal symptoms and detoxification of the body. It would not be wise to start the diet at a time when you are extremely busy and cannot rest normally.

The first couple of days are very crucial. This is the time that the body is trying to heal itself. It is important to remember that the more your body needs a reboot, the more symptoms you'll go through. It is important to track your weight loss progress day by day, and do not go on an all liquid diet for too many days even if you are losing weight very quickly. Staying on a liquid diet for too many days can cause health problems, thus do not adhere to the idea that if something is working for you, you should keep doing it. Things could quickly turn sour. Stick to the diet diligently and patiently and you should see immediate results. Once your body gets used to the change in metabolism, it will start to work on burning those calories and you will lose those extra pounds very fast.

The process of preparing and starting the body reset does not have to be hard at all. It is helpful if your attitude is positive and you go through the process in a manner that is organized. The hardest thing people face is their own motivation, especially first the first few days.

However, once they start seeing the change in their weight it is a huge morale booster! Remember to always keep your end goal in mind and work hard towards it. Once you manage to get through the hard part, the weight loss and your spike in energy will have you feeling great.

Before you start your reset, make sure you have an assortment of ingredients that will help you in the process of making the smoothies and your meals. Some of these foods will be new to you so plan your routine ahead. Before starting the body reset, you should try all the recipes you have picked for various smoothies and see how you like them. Since that is all you will be consuming for the next five days, you better be sure that you know what you are making.

Not enjoying what you eat/drink is one of the biggest reasons why people drop out from different diet regimen. When you're investing your health in fresh products, try and buy organic vegetables and fruits instead.

Organic health is great for eliminating toxins and chemicals from your body. Furthermore, organic fruits and vegetables taste better.

When going on a body reset, try to make your smoothies as fresh as possible. The minute any fresh juice or smoothie hits the air, it starts to oxidize and gradually starts to loss all the nutrients. To get the most out of your smoothies, have them fresh. If that means waking up ten minutes earlier in the morning, so be it!

Your commitment should be to your diet and the more dedicated you are, the better the result you will get out of this diet. However, do not forget to always clean your blender thoroughly after each use. The residue that is left behind becomes a breeding ground for various bacteria. Clean your machine every day without compromise, after each use, no matter how many times a day you use it.

If the idea of just abruptly starting the body reset seems difficult to you, you can make the process easier by trying the following tips. Three days before the starting date, switch to a light diet that is healthy. Give up all unhealthy food and cut down or avoid alcohol, caffeine, red meat, sugar, and gluten. This helps lessen the food cravings that can occur when you first start the diet. Try and consume whole grains and fresh fruits and vegetables.

If you feel you already have a healthy lifestyle then this process can be skipped altogether. However, before you start the diet itself, set yourself up for success. Set an attitude that is positive. It will help motivate you for the diet ahead. First of all, make the intention to start on whatever date you decide. This intention is your commitment to the decision you've made to alter what is unhealthy about your lifestyle and what you feel you need to change. Keep your goal in mind; reflect on it, and also how many pounds you are looking to lose and the changes you are hoping to see. It all just depends on one's own dedication and commitment.

5: The Diet Plan – What To Shop For

The basic idea of the diet plan is simple. Five days on smoothies only and two snacks. The next 5 days you swap one smoothie with a meal. The 5 days after, you swap another smoothie with a meal, slowly adjusting back to your normal routine after 15 days. It may sound pretty simple but to prepare a nutritious smoothie several times a day that fulfills your bodily needs is in itself not a simple task.

Also, adapting to totally new low-calorie meals can be a challenge and you might feel lost as to where to even start. Well, this is how it is supposed to be done. First and foremost, get a shopping list ready so you have your pantry stocked whenever you need to make yourself a meal. For dieters who are starting the body reset plan, here a few things that should definitely be on your shopping list.

First and foremost, a good quality blender is a must. It may sound pretty obvious, but if you're going on an all-liquid diet for about five days you need to make sure your equipment doesn't give up on you.

PEARS AND APPLE

According to a Brazilian study, women who consumed the most pears and apples lost more weight compared to those who ate them the least. Additionally, these fruits help boost your immune system, and they're delicious!

BLUEBERRIES AND RASPBERRIES

Berries are the ultimate super food and they help in cutting down on belly fat according to a study conducted by the University of Michigan. These fruits are also super rich in anti-oxidants so they must be part of your weight loss regimen.

CHIA SEEDS

These are an excellent source of fiber, calcium, and omega 3 fatty acids. Chia seeds are a great when it comes to weight loss. The fiber and protein will make you feel less hungry because they are rich in antioxidants.

Furthermore, they are also capable of absorbing various toxins from the digestive system. If you prefer creamier smoothie, you can even use chia seed gel. Either way, it is an absolutely essential component of your smoothie.

CINNAMON

Cinnamon not only helps lower blood pressure, but it also makes you more alert. It also helps regulate the sugar levels in the blood by improving the metabolism of glucose. If you are worried about abdominal fat, then cinnamon is known to be most effective method in getting rid of belly fat. Use it in your smoothies to enhance taste as well as nutrition.

FAT-FREE, PLAIN GREEK YOGURT

Ongoing research now claims that a dairy-rich diet can actually help promote weight loss. So add some fat-free yogurt to your pantry to make some delicious smoothies.

LIMES AND ORANGES

Citrus fruits are low in calories and help aid digestion as well as boosting the immune system since it is rich in vitamin C. In addition, oranges contain hesperidin, which is a phytonutrient that helps reduce cholesterol and blood pressure.

PROTEIN POWDER

An adequate protein intake is absolutely essential especially when you are on a diet as it helps build keep muscles healthy. A little additional protein in your smoothie will be a great benefit.

SPINACH

This iron-loaded, nutritious vegetable only contains seven calories per cup. Spinach helps in digestion due to its high fiber content and it also slows down aging process. It even aids in building healthy bones.

AVOCADO

Avocados are highly recommended as part of your weight loss. They help thicken the smoothie and give the smoothie the creaminess that it deserves. Additionally, they are a great source of healthy fat that is needed for balanced nutrition. Also, it keeps those pesky hunger cravings away until it's time for the next meal.

CAYENNE PEPPER

This spice adds a little something extra to the smoothie and helps boost your capability to lose weight. According to research, by adding cayenne pepper to your breakfast, you reduce your intake of fat and carbohydrates later in the day. To state it simply, adding cayenne pepper to your food helps reign in your appetite.

LEAFY GREEN

Even though spinach has been mentioned separately, incorporating other leafy greens such as kale, dandelion and lettuce are a big plus. Additionally, all of them contain phytonutrients that are high in fiber.

PULP FROM DIFFERENT FRUITS

If you are using a juicer to extract juices to add to various smoothies, there is a lot of pulp leftover from the juicing process. This pulp consists mostly of fiber that was separated from the fruit juice. Instead of throwing it out, you may add it to your smoothies instead for increased fiber intake.

TEA/ICE/WATER

Even though it all mainly depends on the different recipes that you use, many recipes require fruit juice or milk to be added to the smoothie so that it can come out right consistently. However, to get rid of the extra calories (if you feel that your calorie intake is too high), you may add water, tea or just ice instead. Green tea is already very popular for its various health benefits and cleansing properties, thus it can be a perfect substitute in case you do not want to add milk or juice. Green tea is also great for weight loss and is known to be very effective.

THINGS TO AVOID

While there are a variety of foods that give a wonderful flavor to your smoothies without adding any extra calories, there are also some pitfalls. Smoothies are a very nutritious and healthy option, which they are indeed, but they can also be fattening.

There are some ingredients that you need to steer away from when you are trying to lose weight. Excess sugar in smoothies should be avoided. Even natural sugar from honey or maple syrup should be kept to a minimum in an effort to reduce calorie counts.

CANNED VEGETABLES AND FRUITS

Fresh produce is always the most effective and healthy option when it comes to diet. However, in case you can't find specific fruits that you want to incorporate, than it is much better to turn to frozen foods or leave the ingredient out totally rather than picking canned vegetables or fruits. These cans contain numerous preservatives and also artificial sweeteners that just make them all the more fattening.

The processing that canned fruit undergoes also causes it to lose out on the bulk of nutrients and vitamins that the fruit originally had. Frozen and fresh fruits and vegetables are able to maintain their nutritional value and contents for over a longer period of time compared to canned goods.

DAIRY

While there are certain exceptions to this rule such as Greek Yogurt or raw milk, dairy products are full of calories, and thus it is preferable that they are avoided. However, frozen yogurt, ice cream, milk and other dairy products are usually quite a common component of smoothies. Greek yogurt however, is low in sugar but has high protein content and thus it is recommended.

FRUIT EXTRACT OR JUICE

Fruit Juice itself is usually very high in sugar even though these natural sugars are much healthier than the processed sugar in our usual diet. However, if one is looking to lose weight then fruit juice should ideally be avoided or should be monitored. Store-bought fruit juices are even worse as they lose most of their nutritional value as bottled juice undergoes pasteurization. They also contain additional artificial sweeteners and contain zero fiber. A small amount of fruit juice in a limited amount is okay, but too much of it will just increase the calorie intake and impede weight loss.

PROTEIN POWDERS

This may come as a surprise as this very product was mentioned before as something one SHOULD invest in. In some cases it might actually not be a very good idea. Protein powders are good for people who want to bulk up and add muscle mass. However, for pure weight loss purposes, it would be better to stick to natural sources of proteins like grains, nuts etc. In the body reset diet, since the first five days consist of smoothies only, protein powder is recommended to fulfill daily requirements.

SWEETENERS

The worst thing you can do is consume too much sugar by over-sweetening your smoothies. It is the absolute worst thing to do! The high sugar in the diet will be counterproductive as it will delay and suppress the metabolic reboot. Stevia is a natural sweetener with no calories that can be substituted for sugar.

EXCESS OF SWEET FRUIT

While fresh and whole fruits are an excellent way to add natural flavor to your smoothies along with a little sweetness, it is important to remember to keep a balance since too much of it can be a serious problem. Too much fruit in just a single smoothie can cause your blood sugar levels to shoot and may also cause various problems with digestion. A valuable rule of thumb to abide by is to stick to berries and avocados. However, it is fine to incorporate small amounts of sweet fruits like apples, bananas, pineapples, or mangoes, but it must be kept to a bare minimum preferably. Smoothies with too much sugar will give the exact opposite result of what we want. Instead, they are a perfect recipe to gain weight rather than to lose weight.

Once you've stocked up on basic ingredients for PHASE 1 you can successfully experiment and create your own smoothies if you're feeling creative. However, try and stick to low calories and for the first few days. It'll be best to adhere to tested weight loss recipes rather than creating your own. Ideally you should be having a 'white' smoothie in the morning, a 'red' smoothie for lunch and a 'green' smoothie for dinner.

Additionally, you need to be having two crunchy snacks too. For example, an apple, or a tablespoon of almond batter with three crackers etc. If you stick to this plan with dedication, you should lose weight drastically just by the end of phase 1 alone.

6: Recipes

To give you a head start regarding the sort of smoothies you can create, here are some easy to make delicious recipes for you to follow.

BREAKFAST KING

Take five raw almonds either whole or chopped and add them to a blender. In the blender, add one red apple that hasn't been peeled. It should be chopped up with the core removed. Also, add one chopped frozen banana, three-fourth of a cup of plain Greek yogurt, half a cup of fat-free milk, and half a teaspoon of cinnamon. Blend this all together and you have a delicious breakfast drink!

RED POISON (LUNCH)

In a blender, add a cup of frozen raspberries, one-fourth of a cup of frozen blueberries, and half an orange that has been peeled. Then add three-fourth cup of Greek yogurt, half a cup of either water, almond milk, or skimmed milk, and a table spoon of ground walnuts or flaxseeds. Blend and enjoy

GREEN ENVY (DINNER)

Blend together two cups of spinach leaves, one unpeeled ripe pear that has been chopped with the core removed, fifteen grapes (green or red depends on your taste), three fourth cup of plain Greek yogurt, two tablespoons of chopped avocados, a tablespoon of lime juice and half a cup of either water, almond milk or skim milk. This makes a delicious green mixture that you can enjoy at the end of the day.

PINA COLADA

Blend together one peeled orange, one-third cup of coconut milk and a scoop of whey protein powder. Also, add one banana that has been cut into chunks and a cup of pineapple chunks. Blend it together to make a delicious creamy Pina Colada.

PERFECT WEIGHT LOSS SMOOTHIE

Blend together:
One cup of water
Half an avocado (medium sized)
Half a cup of fresh or frozen blueberries
Half a tablespoon of honey or maple syrup
Half a tablespoon of coconut oil
A tablespoon of chia seeds
Chill in the refrigerator. Serve it cold.

MANGO GREEN TEA SMOOTHIE

Blend together a cup of green tea, one cup of frozen or fresh mango chunks, half avocado, half tablespoon of coconut oil, one cup of spinach, a little bit of sea salt to taste and a little bit of honey, stevia or maple syrup if you want to sweeten it up a bit more. This makes a delicious low calorie sweet drink.

BANANA BERRY SMOOTHIE

Blend together a cup of water, half a banana that has been chopped into chunks, a cup of fresh berries (mixed), one cup of spinach, a tablespoon of coconut oil, one fourth teaspoon of cayenne pepper, and one tablespoon of gelatin for additional protein if needed. This is a perfect instant energy drink that restores alertness and energy levels instantly.

STRAWBERRY KIWI SMOOTHIE

To make this green smoothie, take two cups of baby arugula, two kiwifruit that have been chopped and peeled, five fresh strawberries, one frozen chopped banana and two tablespoons of soy protein. You can even increase the fiber content by adding the skins of different fruits such as apples, pears, and peaches. However, do not add the kiwi fruit unpeeled because the skin is tough and cannot be blended.

LEMON RASPBERRY SMOOTHIE

Take a cup of frozen raspberries, three tablespoons of lemon juice, three fourth cup of ice chips, six ounces of Greek yogurt and twelve raw cashew nuts. Blend all these together to a consistency that you prefer. Voila!

STONE FRUIT SMOOTHIE

For this recipe you need to mix together in a blender two chopped peaches without the core, one chopped apricot, cup of frozen or preferably fresh strawberries and also about six ounces of plain fat free Greek yoghurt. Also, add to the blender about two tablespoons of ground flaxseeds and one cup of small ice chip or ice cubes whichever are available. Blend this all together to the consistency that you desire and this makes for an absolutely delicious smoothie.

PEANUT BUTTER & JELLY SMOOTHIE

All of your favorite flavors in a sandwich are combined together in one delicious smoothie. To make this smoothie, you need two cups of frozen or preferably fresh strawberries, add one chopped frozen banana, add two teaspoons of peanut butter and about half a cup of ice chips or cubes. Finally, you can also add four ounces of plain fat free yogurt, and blend it all together. This is a delicious smoothie you can add to your lunch menu.

Now that you have a wide assortment of smoothies, you can easily choose the ones you'd prefer to get you through the body reset. These delicious concoctions are filling and packed with energy. However, no matter how much you like the taste, do not have more smoothies than you are supposed to as it will be counterproductive.

Once you move on to phase two, you need to incorporate some solid food back into your diet. The food should ideally be mostly natural and must stay around 300-350 calories. It isn't a good idea to eat more than that.

However, as long as you stay within the nutritional guidelines and eat healthy, there is no restriction on the sort of solid food you may incorporate back in your diet. Some good examples are hummus, couscous, sandwiches etc. As long as you're eating in your calorie limit and eating healthy food, you can explore whatever meal options you prefer.

Once you start reaching the end of the diet, you will not only see how much weight you have managed to lose but you will also feel immense satisfaction for accomplishing your goals. Apart from the weight loss, the detoxification and high energy levels will leave you feeling absolutely amazing!

7: Exercise, Routines, and Sleep Patterns

It is not just about what you eat that determines weight loss. Resetting your body systems also means getting plenty of exercise, changing your daily routine and getting plenty of sleep. All these factors contribute to body reset diet and weight loss.

When it comes to exercise during the body reset diet, training hours at the gym and heavy exercise isn't actually recommended. When cutting down on calories, too much exercise won't be very helpful and might even have you feeling sick and fatigued. Secondly, it also prompts the body to start attempting to conserve calories due to excessive exertion, which means that metabolism rate will go down.

The exercise that is recommended involves one of the easiest ways to get yourself moving: walking. Whether you're outside or just pacing in your own room, walking every day is an adequate exercise while on this diet. If you really want to add more exercise to the agenda, you can add light resistance training without weights.

There is no need for heavy-duty exercise. However, there is some resistance training you can do two to three times a week. This will set you up for long term weight loss. These exercises include crunches, squats, and push-ups.

CRUNCHES

Your form is the most important thing when doing crunches. Lie on your back and bend your knees. Keep your feet flat on the floor. Then, place your hands behind your head and slightly place your chin down slightly. While doing so just lift your shoulders and head off the exercise mat, and make sure that you are involving your core muscles in this exercise. Continue lifting yourself and curling up and make sure the upper back is well off the mat. Keep the position for a short while and then gently lower the torso back. Repeat this circuit.

STANDARD PUSH-UPS

This is a classic exercise that everyone should know how to do. It is very effective as it involves a wide range of muscle groups.

SQUAT

Stand straight ensuring that your feet are either parallel or they are turned about fifteen degrees or whatever pose you feel comfortable maintaining. Then, slowly begin to crouch down behind your knees and the hips until your thighs are at least parallel to the floor. You have to make sure that the heels do not rise above the floor. Return back to your standing position by pressing through the heels.

BURPEES

This is one of the most effective exercises that involve the entire body. First, set yourself in a squat position but your hands must be on the floor. After this, push your feet back as if you're about to do a push-up and complete one push-up. However, after completing the push-up, promptly return back to the squat position. Jump up as high as you can before squatting again and then go back into the push up position of this exercise.

PLANK

This exercise engages the abdominal muscles the most. First, you must lie with your face down, and your forearm has to be on the floor with your hands clasped together. Basically, you are supporting your body weight on your fore-arms. Gradually, extend your legs far behind your body and then rise up on your toes. Make sure that your back is absolutely straight. Follow this by tightening your core and hold this position for at least thirty to sixty seconds or as long as you can manage.

You should do these exercises three a week. For beginners, they can begin with less number of circuits but for people who are big on exercise, their workout should be slightly more prolonged and extensive.

There are other things that you can do to train your body to control hunger, hormones, banish cravings, and boost the metabolism. Apart from just resetting the metabolism of the body, you should reset your internal body clock that controls your sleeping and eating patterns.

Once it is set properly, you can tune into the body's natural schedule and get rid of the extra pounds! When you first wake up in the morning, acquire a habit of doing a light exercise before breakfast. Research has proven that people who exercise before breakfast lose weight much more quickly and their metabolic system is much more efficient.

Drink lots and lots of water. Try drinking about three liters of water a day. Research have shown that people who drink two glasses of water before every meal tend to lose almost 5 pounds more than people who don't.

When you wake up, the internal alarm clock also signals the production of 'ghrelin', which is produced in the stomach. This hormone is also called the 'feed me' hormone as it is what signals hunger. If you ignore it, then it is produced even more, making you even hungrier. Thus, after exercising, have your breakfast within an hour of waking up.

Have a light snack about 10 to 11 AM because that is when ghrelin starts produce again. Have a light snack. Have your lunch around 12 to 1 PM. Usually at this time the body tends to produce galanin, a hormone that makes the body crave fat. The higher the body's fat intake, the more galanin is produced. Thus, instead of having fats at this time, it is best to have proteins and some carbohydrates instead.

Ideally, taking a fifteen to twenty minute mid-day nap is perfect. It will give your body a boost and will help you sleep better at night. Instead of going to the vending machines at work and eating an unhealthy snack, go to your car instead for a quick nap.

If you need a caffeine boost, do not take one after 9 o'clock. Taking caffeine late at night disturbs your normal body rhythm and will keep you awake all night.

Have an early dinner around five to seven pm. Add a little bit of healthy fat so you don't wake up at night feeling hungry. Avocados and flaxseed are both good options for healthy fat intake. Around 9 pm, have the second small snack. It should ideally be carbohydrate-based.

A small dose of carbohydrates before bed create tryptophan, which in turn aids the brain in the production of serotonin. Serotonin is a feel-good hormone that helps the body in melatonin production, which helps you fall asleep. Another important thing you have to do after the bed time snack is to turn off digital devices. Step away from them, especially the television. These devices are terribly disruptive and mess up the normal sleep cycle of the body. Do something relaxing instead like taking a bath or reading. Set up a fixed time to wake up and fall asleep every night. A regular cycle helps you fall asleep faster and keeps the body systems in check.

Constant light exposure not only disrupts the sleeping patterns, but it also increases the risk of gaining weight, which is why it is so important to fix this cycle. Constant exposure to light also decreases the production of melatonin, the sleep hormone.

According to research, mice that had normal exposure to light gained fifty percent less weigh than the mice exposed to more light constantly. Thus, when sleeping, darken your room with shades and curtains and try to keep the room as dark as possible during the night. Also wear a sleep mask to try and keep the light out.

The body reset is a whole lifestyle change that will help you set up your whole system on track. This in turn promotes weight loss and helps you stay fit!

8: Obstacles and Advice

As with any other dietary change, there are some bumps along the way that need tweaking and solving. Just a little bit of adjustment can go a long way.

First of all, you need to understand that body reset diet is to help you lose weight, but the main goal is to make you feel good about yourself. So while on this diet you might at times feel the need to cheat and have an unhealthy snack instead. It's best to be prepared for this possibility.

Always have quick snacks handy so you can eat them every time you feel a moment of weakness so you can starve off your cravings. Before you start this diet, you should clean out your entire house and get rid of all the junk food. Make sure there is nothing around that is unhealthy for you. If there is no junk food around, it will break your willpower, and then this whole process will be much easier for you.

However, do remember that if you do end up cheating and you did something you weren't supposed to, do not lose hope! Most people feel so disappointed with themselves in such situations that they abandon their diet altogether and just accept total failure. Well, that is NOT the right way to go about it. If you cheat, then don't berate yourself.

Get rid of the unhealthy food you just snacked on and just throw it out! Once you start seeing results, you will automatically be more motivated to adhere to the entire plan and not give in.

Before you begin your body rest diet, it is best if you talk to your friends and family and tell them beforehand about the diet. Having people supporting you goes a long, long way.

More importantly, it can be very disheartening if you're trying to make a dietary change and a friend shows up at your doorstep with cupcakes or pizza. So it's best to let those friends know beforehand what you are planning to do and you would appreciate the support. Also, some of your friends might even try to convince you not to bother with some diet plan thinking that it may be unhealthy for you.

Terms like 'detox' and 'body reset' do tend to receive skepticism. You can assure your loved ones that you know what you're doing and it isn't unhealthy at all. The best thing to do is just ask for respect, however, don't try and convince others to join you! No two people are alike so while you might feel a diet is appropriate for you, someone else might have a totally opposite opinion about it

DOS AND DON'TS:

- Do not take alcohol on this diet. It is strictly forbidden for fifteen days you are on it.

- Don't stress out! Increase levels of stress result in the production of a hormone called cortisol. This hormone prevents muscle gain and will slow down the weight loss process. So if you're going to keep worrying about your diet and how much weight you are or aren't losing, you're probably just ruining your own chances of this diet being successful. Find different ways to manage your stress. This is supposed to be a time of healing and detoxification of the body.

- Last but not the least, trust the process and the diet. Be patient and be kind to yourself through this journey. If you stick to it, it will prepare you for a whole lifetime of success!

Conclusion

The Body Reset Diet Plan, unlike other diet plans, provides you with a concise cheat sheet to re-wiring your entire system for successful weight loss. Instead of starving yourself and subjecting your body to drastic changes in routine, this diet gives you a perfect system that gives your body the much-needed change that you wanted to see.

The body reset plan also helps improve your sleeping, eating patterns and just about everything the body regulates. Undertaking this diet plan may seem like quite a task but in the end as the saying goes, "the proof is in the pudding." Once you start seeing results, it will definitely make you feel more confident about own yourself and the efficacy of this diet.